C000061113

Printed in the United Kingdom.

First Printing, 2015

ISBN 13: 978-1-84481-000-0

ISBN 10: 1-84481-000-3

Warning and Disclaimer

Although every precaution has been taken to verify the accuracy of
the information contained herein, the author and publisher assume
no responsibility for any errors or omissions. No liability is assumed
for damage or injury that may result from the use of information
contained within.

Fighter's Codex

D. Amerland

Introduction

Fighter's Codex is a martial art style training program for general fitness. It is a high intensity workout regimen that will streamline and tone and give your body strength and agility. It's 100% no-equipment and home friendly program. It is suitable for a beginner and it will work for a pro, too. You will practice kicks and punches, work on your flexibility and balance and even learn some fighting techniques while getting fit. From a training point of view it will physically transform you to a martial artist. If you already do some martial arts it will take you to an entirely new level in 30 days.

The Fighter's Codex is a forge. It will take the raw power that is "you" and, over 30 days, turn it into a highly efficient, potentially lethal, kick-ass, fighting machine. You could be new to this or you may already be doing some martial art, it's designed to benefit you regardless. Go through each day, pick a level (where appropriate) and follow through the exercises. If you're not sure about the execution of any of them check out the videos in our exercise library.

There are performance, practice and recuperation days all built into this. It is designed to increase your speed, stamina, strength, flexibility, tendon strength and motor-coordination skills. You will perform some of the training routines practiced by world class martial artists. It will make you aware of your body and the way it moves in a way you have never quite been before. There are also handy, instructional videos you can access on the Darebee.com YouTube channel that better illustrate some techniques.

Those who go through it get to meet their badass self on the other side of the 30 days.

Guide to Punching

The hand is probably the most versatile part of our body. Tool and weapon in equal parts it is no surprise to discover that it has actually evolved, over thousands of years, to form a punch and hit a target. Sure, its shape and opposable thumb give it dexterity that allows us to do things like work a wrench and play the guitar but, the argument goes, there are several different possible variations in its proportion that could allow us to do that, but only one that would allow it to be both tool and weapon.

To understand exactly why all you have to do is clench your fist hard and look at the back of it from above. What do you feel and what do you notice? As you clench your fist tightly you can actually feel all the delicate bones of your hand pulling tightly together. The tendons shortening so that the fist suddenly becomes harder as a structure, more stable. Then, as you look at the back of your closed fist from above you notice that not all knuckles are equal. The knuckle that's at the base of your index finger (also known as the second meta-carpo-phalangeal (MCP), sticks out a little more than the rest.

The effect is known as buttressing (support) and the way the knuckles stick out when the hand is clenched hard to form a tight fist, along with the shortening of all the other tendons is designed to increase the punching power of the fist at the point of impact while protecting the delicate bones of the hand.

A study carried out by researchers Utah showed that while the amount of power delivered to a target with the open palm is the same as that delivered with a clenched fist the amount of measurable power delivered at the point of impact per square millimeters of surface increased considerably. It also doubled the ability of the proximal phalanges (the bones of the fingers that articulate with the MCP joints) to transmit a punching force.

The increase in power delivered is understandable. As the surface area we strike with shrinks the amount of power that goes through it also increases. It's a bit like having your foot stepped on by accident by 150lb person wearing sneakers and then the same person stepping on you accidentally wearing high heeled boots. The pain you will experience and the damage you will suffer when the latter happens is amplified manifold because the force that is applied is now concentrated on a very small area of your foot.

When it came to punching however what was surprising in regards was that the clenched fist strengthened the ability of the bones connected to the knuckles to transmit punching force which means that with our fists clenched we simply strike harder because we know we can strike harder and get damaged less.

This also explains why boxers wrap their hands before they put on boxing gloves. A good handwrap tightens up around the hand when the fist is clenched adding extra buttressing and allows the boxer to strike harder without running the risk of injuring his hands.

So, now that we know that our hands evolved to be these incredible weapons, how do we actually use them to maximum advantage?

How to Form a Fist

While most of us know how to form a fist, understanding the reasons behind a proper fist will help us avoid making mistakes that lead to injuries. The principle of forming a proper fist can be summarized in one word: alignment. Basically you want to make sure that everything is aligned both internally and externally to allow you to deliver the maximum striking force, safely.

You can transform your hands from delicate instruments to powerful weapons in four easy steps:

1. Hold your hand out like you would for a handshake, palm open, thumb pointing towards the ceiling.
2. Now fold the extended fingers of your hand towards the center of your palm, but keep your thumb pointing towards the ceiling. Make sure that your fingertips are buried in the middle of your palm.
3. Now fold your thumb in tightly, over your fingers, until the ball of your thumb touches the middle joint of your index finger (called interphalangeal joint or IP for short). You now have a perfectly

formed fist, but we are not finished yet.

4. Next, turn your hand ninety degrees so that your thumb is looking

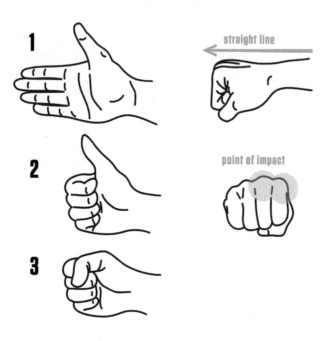

towards the ground. Make sure that there is a perfectly straight line between your forearm and the end of your fist. To test this hold your arm perfectly straight in front of you and check to see that this is indeed so by sighting along it. You will most probably have to move your hand slightly downwards to achieve that and then, slightly outwards to make sure that its most prominent point when it's in a clenched fist are the first two knuckle joints.

That's it. You now have formed not just the perfect fist but also have aligned the muscles of the forearm and the tendons of the wrist and have made sure that the metacarpal bone and the delicate bones of the fingers are protected from stress fractures and impact damage, respectively. The tightness of the fist also protects the bones of the hand from the stress forces that are generated when we punch.

PUNCHING
FORM

DAREBEE
PUNCHING GUIDE
© darebee.com

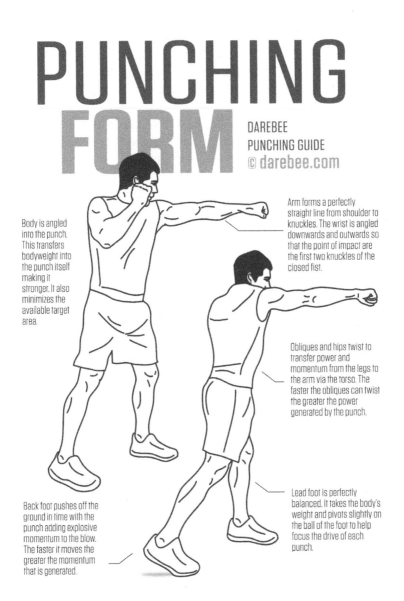

Body is angled into the punch. This transfers bodyweight into the punch itself making it stronger. It also minimizes the available target area.

Arm forms a perfectly straight line from shoulder to knuckles. The wrist is angled downwards and outwards so that the point of impact are the first two knuckles of the closed fist.

Obliques and hips twist to transfer power and momentum from the legs to the arm via the torso. The faster the obliques can twist the greater the power generated by the punch.

Back foot pushes off the ground in time with the punch adding explosive momentum to the blow. The faster it moves the greater the momentum that is generated.

Lead foot is perfectly balanced. It takes the body's weight and pivots slightly on the ball of the foot to help focus the drive of each punch.

the arms of cadavers found that when we have a properly formed fist we can punch with twice the force than if we used the open palm.

Punching Technique

Forming the perfect fist is only half the battle of course. We also need to know how to punch. Here the variations are a lot broader and range from the rapid-fire short punches of Kung-Fu to the hip-thrown, twisting punches of Karate and the structurally strong cross and hook punches of Boxing.

There are two things to remember here that are important. First, that all punches are designed to do the same thing: get the clenched first that is at the end of our arm to a target that is within reach of us. Second, not all punches are intended to have the same effect. Some punches are considered harder than others for reasons we will get to later. Some punches are finishing punches intended to knock an opponent out or damage him significantly while other punches are sounding punches, used to keep an opponent busy and create an opening for a stronger, follow-up attack. The difference between each is in what we call 'structure' which we will also cover a little further down.

Irrespective of which punch you decide to throw or what you intend it to do two things will hold fast. First, there will be some sort of twisting motion taking place as your fist goes from a position where the inside of your wrist is facing you (or looking to your side) to one where your arm is outstretched, the forearm and wrist aligned and perfect straight, the two front knuckles the foremost striking point. Second, the power of your punch will always depend upon the amount of bodyweight you have been able to move and the speed you have been able to move it at, while punching.

A truly powerful punch is the haymaker which looks a little like someone throwing a shotput, except they throw a punch instead. It rarely works however because despite its power it is such an obvious punch with so much body movement and a long travelling distance that it is easy to evade. There is little purpose in throwing a punch if it is so obvious that it will never connect with its intended target.

Every punching technique then tries to find the optimal distance between ourselves and the target while still holding the arms back enough to allow for some travelling distance and the building up of power and deliver it at sufficient speed to actually hit the target before it escapes. That means that the nearer we have placed our fists to a target the softer the punch is going to be. The exception to this rule is Bruce Lee's famous one-inch punch which we shall return to below.

So, in order for a punch to be strong it needs to:

Engage as many muscle groups as possible. Aligned muscle groups add to and amplify each other's strength. In the early days of boxing, boxers fought with bare knuckles. To protect their hands from damage they kept their clenched fists in front of them, with the inside of the forearm facing them and they flicked them out towards the opponent, using the first two, prominent knuckles to strike with. This is a movement that uses the biceps and shoulder and flicks the arm out as the elbow joint opens and closes. It is therefore a relatively weak punch. Modern boxers hold their fists in front of them, usually with the inside of the forearms facing each other and they twist their arms when they punch. This engages the deltoid, trapezius, triceps, elbow joint, forearm muscles and wrist tendons making the punch way harder and that's before we even consider the bodyweight that is added to this by the rotation and commitment of the upper body, through the pelvic girdle muscles and the contribution made to the movement by quads and calves.

Employ as much of the body's weight as possible. This is pure physics. The more of the body's weight that can be placed 'behind' the punch the heavier that punch will be. This is also why heavier people have naturally harder punches.

Use as much push off the ground as possible. If you are suspended in space or floating in water it is impossible to punch hard. That's because of Newton's third law of motion which states that every action has an equal and opposite reaction. When you punch hard and you are suspended in midair (or in water) the same force with which you punch, is also pushed back into your own body. Without your legs being connected to the ground and pushing off it, there is no way to generate any meaningful force in the direction that you are punching towards.

What makes a punch powerful?

When it comes to having powerful punches physics again kicks in. Power is mass x acceleration. A powerful punch is always a combination of how quickly the arm will move, how much of the body's weight can be committed to the punch by pushing off the ground with the legs and how all this is synchronized.

Usually the longer a punch travels to reach its target the greater acceleration it can achieve and the more commitment in terms of the body's weight can be placed behind it. That's why the boxer's jab, delivered with the hand nearest the opponent is fast but cannot be very powerful while the cross, which is delivered by the hand held further back is always way more powerful as a blow.

One exception to this very obvious rule is Bruce Lee's famous one-inch punch which we mentioned earlier in the article. Bruce Lee trained himself to synchronize his muscles and move his body explosively when he punched. So although he was about an inch away from his target (which is where the punch gets its name from) he was still able to deliver a heavy blow thanks to the acceleration of his whole body that he could achieve. Because Bruce Lee had trained himself to synchronize of all his muscles so that the power generated from his legs could travel up his torso and explode in his fist and the commitment of his body he was able to generate a lot of power using the mass x acceleration equation, of physics.

Basically he was able to move his entire body very explosively which made his punches way heavier than they should realistically have been.

Here are the elements which make a punch powerful:

- Strong legs – to help push off the ground
- Strong abdominals – to help transmit the power from the legs to the upper torso
- Good upper body strength – to help punch hard and fast in the

first instance

To see how this works we will consider here a straight punch, as opposed to a hook or an uppercut or a backfist. A straight punch like the jab or the cross are very common punches and amongst the easiest to throw. It is powered by:

- Deltoids
- Triceps
- Chest
- Trapezius

Boxers do a lot of push ups and pulls ups which strengthen these muscles so they can have stronger punches. But then they also do a lot of squats, running, jogging, sprinting and skipping as well as ab work.

To truly make a punch hard beyond strong punch delivery muscles, they also need:

- **Strong quads** – to power their upper body as it twists into the punch.
- **Powerful calves** – to push off the ground.
- **Great abs** – to smoothly transfer power from the lower body to the upper one.

Plus because a punch, as we saw above relies on mass and acceleration a really strong punch also requires:

- **Good limb speed** – the arms have to be able to move explosively fast.
- **Explosive leg work** – heavy hitters are able to push off the ground with their calves really fast.

This principle of a powerful punch is the same regardless if you are looking at, let's say a boxer's cross or a martial artist's traditional hip punch. While the boxer requires a more upper body commitment with his cross punch, the martial artist requires a greater torso rotation with his hips in order to power the hip punch.

11

This is where we get the notion of 'structure' in punches. Essentially, a punch is made up of all the muscle groups that are recruited in order to power it. A quick jab for example may only make use of three muscle groups (Deltoids, Triceps and Chest muscles) and it is relatively a structurally weak punch. A hook on the other hand may use Deltoids, Triceps, Biceps, Lats, Abs, Glutes, Quads and Calves all of which make it a structurally stronger punch. The more structurally strong a punch is the harder it is to defend against. A jab, for example may be blocked but a hook needs to be evaded.

Benefits of Training with Punches

Because punches recruit so many muscle groups learning to throw a proper punch is a great way of getting fit. Shadow boxing, for example, where multiple punches are thrown at an imaginary target in midair is a great way to condition the muscles and improve aerobic fitness and increase endurance.

One of the most common complaints voiced by beginners is that they fail to feel anything much when they throw punches. That is to be expected for three reasons:

First, in the beginning punching muscles are relatively weak and have not been trained so there is not a lot of muscular activity going on when punches are thrown.

Second, because it's early stages there is not a lot of synchronization going on in the muscle groups so punching feels both easy and not very powerful.

Third, the lower body is not yet engaged at this stage.

All of these come later. The more you throw punches the stronger your arms and shoulders get and the stronger they get, the more muscles they begin to engage. So basically repetitive punching is one of the most tried and tested ways of building punching power by gradually increasing the structural makeup of the punches we throw.

If along with the punching we also add some footwork like bouncing on the spot and moving from side to side then we will find that we get a total workout just by shadow boxing for twenty minutes.

This is the kind of physical activity that builds lean, functional, powerful muscles, increases endurance and improves aerobic performance.

If you happen to have a heavy bag around you can also put it to good use to help you develop powerful punches. While shadow boxing is great for developing punching speed and great form, a heavy bag helps in developing structurally powerful punches and synchronized muscles. The heavy bag absorbs the force of each blow and sends a powerful feedback wave travelling back up the muscles of the arm, shoulder, back an abs. This doubles the load of the workout on your arms and body and introduces a heavy endurance component to your training.

Heavy bag training is great for building strength, denser, harder-working muscles and improving balance, coordination, aerobic performance and endurance.

Training for Stronger Punches

If we are serious about increasing the power of our punches and also, in the process, taking our fitness to a new level we need to:

- Do fast, deep push-ups, engaging the triceps, chest, deltoids and trapezium muscles in full motion, explosive movements.
- Do fast, full-motion sit ups.
- Work our obliques with twisting sit ups and our core with planks.
- Work our glutes with squats and work our lower back with back extensions.
- Work our quads with squats and work out calves with skipping rope and bouncing on the spot.

At the same time we will need to do some running to help all these different muscles work smoothly together.

When we see just how many muscles are involved in punching we begin to understand why boxers command such respect and have such structurally strong (i.e. heavy) punches and why it takes so much time and effort to begin to feel the effects and benefits of punching training. When we can throw a structurally strong punch however, we also have the means to exercise and get fit no matter where we are.

Guide to Kicks

Our legs are enormously strong, they are longer than our arms and we use them from the moment we learn how to walk. Kicking however is not easy and there are several reasons for that. In order to do it correctly it requires a great deal of balance and precision. Because the muscles we are using are large, it also requires endurance and kicking can become really tiring, really quickly, unless of course we have trained for it.

That means that like everything else that has to do with physical performance there is a definite skill to kicking well and technique as well as physical conditioning, become important factors.

Given how difficult it is to kick well the primary question must be why do it at all? After all our bodies have adapted fantastically well to fighting in a forward stance, using our two arms and balancing perfectly well on both of our sturdy legs. Why compromise this intuitive mechanism for combat in order to deliver a little more muscle power?

There are several good reasons which we need to keep in mind:

Power. Although we are Apex Predators on our planet, without our technology we are inherently weak. We have muscle-to-mass ratio. Our muscles are acquired rather than inherited. We have no large teeth or claws. What we are really well adapted for is running continuously over very long distances and this is where our legs actually come in as weapons. The reasoning goes that if we can correctly harness their muscle power we suddenly have two very potent weapons to bring into play, if need be.

Reach. Because we are generally weak and vulnerable, close quarter combat does not suit us very well. Our legs are longer than our arms, they can reach a target we are striking without having to get too close to it physically and put ourselves in harm's way.

Strength. Square a man and a woman against each other and the man has a distinct advantage. Men are not only physically larger than

15

Chamber
Position

BY DAREBEE
© darebee.com

Chamber position is the 'cocking form' of the leg prior to firing off a kick. It is formed from either the front or back leg and it is the required stage before you can successfully launch any kick.

Back Arm

Your back arm is there to guard your chin and also launch an attack should you decide not to kick.

Lead Arm

Keep it near your lead knee or a little higher to act as a guard. Its main function is to help your body balance.

Knee

The height you raise your knee to determines the height of your kick. A direct hip-knee-target line of attack is formed by the position.

Hip

The body is arched over the hip so that the weight is carried by the skeleton, rather than the muscles. This way you have greater stability and can maintain this position longer, without tiring.

A raised knee also acts as a guard. This is the position practically every kick gets fired off from.

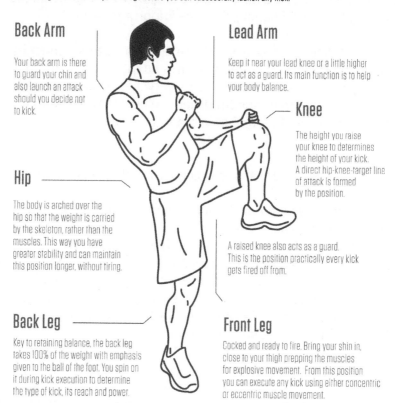

Back Leg

Key to retaining balance, the back leg takes 100% of the weight with emphasis given to the ball of the foot. You spin on it during kick execution to determine the type of kick, its reach and power.

Front Leg

Cocked and ready to fire. Bring your shin in, close to your thigh prepping the muscles for explosive movement. From this position you can execute any kick using either concentric or eccentric muscle movement.

16

women but they also have much greater upper body strength which gives them an advantage in grappling and punching. But that gender difference becomes a lot less noticeable when we get to lower body strength. There a woman can be as

strong as a man, almost, which is why kicking is also a great gender equalizer.

Mobility. It sounds counterintuitive to say that by raising one leg to kick and standing on only one leg you gain mobility but that is actually what can happen. An unarmed combat situation is a highly fluid one where steps being taken are dead time and can also telegraph your intent, making a move obvious and destroying the element of surprise in an attack. By kicking and using the momentum of the kick to also take a step as the foot lands a skilled fighter can gain ground much faster and can either move away from or towards an opponent with minimal downtime.

Kicks and Martial Arts
Kicks, of course, have become synonymous with martial arts but they have been with unarmed combat throughout the ages. They were used by ancient warriors fighting with edged weapons on the battlefield as a means of distracting an opponent or, at times, as a weapon of last resort. And even the brutal (and illegal) bare knuckle street fighting of the past had a "boots and fists" rule, which also was the only rule it seemed to have.

In martial arts kicking has reached an art form. By turning the body itself into a weapon, different styles have contributed different types of kicks, each with its own advantages and disadvantages when it comes to performing them. Some kicks use long, circular motions, others are more direct and others still are a mix of the two. Kicks can be performed statically, from a standing still position. They can be performed while in motion, alone or as part of a two or three kick combination.

While they appear to be different in essence their foundation is the same. Biomechanics and physics dictate that realistically there are only so many ways we can kick and still deliver effective power on a target.

Types of Kicks

Before we mention the six primary types of kicks it's worth remembering that a kick can be delivered either from the front or the back leg. The difference is in speed of delivery vs power and this is where physics comes in. A front leg kick reaches the target you're attacking faster but utilizes less of the body's weight to do so. A kick delivered from the back leg will take longer to reach the target and travel a longer distance to do so but will gain more power in the process and utilize more of the body's weight, making it a harder kick. There is no 'wrong' or 'right' in the choices you make when you kick. The choice each time depends upon your ability, the particular martial art you are trained in and, obviously, what is required by the situation.

Although we will look at six fundamental types of kicks, essentially there are only two types of basic kicks they all spring from: Push kicks and arc kicks.

Push kicks, as the name suggests, utilize the strong leg muscles, bunching them up like a spring and then releasing them in a straight line, to the target. Push kicks have an immediate, powerful effect and are hard to block against. They are fast kicks that generate a lot of power which even if blocked, creates an impact so they can never be ignored. Because they are fast and travel the shortest distance to a target they are also hard to evade.

Arc kicks, as the name suggests, take the leg through a curved trajectory that is necessary for power to be developed. Arc kicks are great for fighting in unorthodox positions (i.e. not facing forward), dealing with multiple opponents at once (when the traditional coiling and uncoiling action of a push kick takes too much time to execute more than a couple of times) or for generating power that is disproportionate in size to the strength of the muscles involved (proving that even physically smaller or weaker opponents can generate powerful kicks).

If you watch a Van Damme film or have ever seen Joe Lewis fight, you'll see that they are both primary proponents of push kicks. Bruce

Types of **Kicks**

by DAREBEE © darebee.com

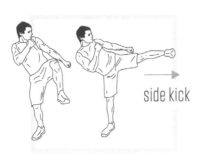

side kick

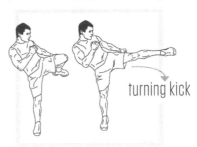

turning kick

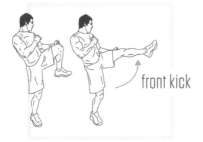

front kick

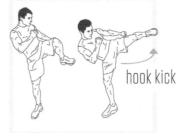

hook kick

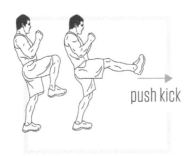

push kick

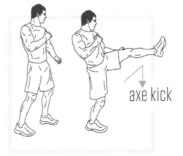

axe kick

The Difference Between
Turning, Side and Hook Kicks

by DAREBEE
© darebee.com

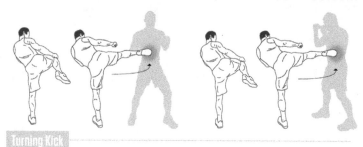

Turning Kick

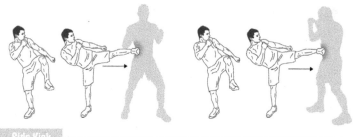

Side Kick

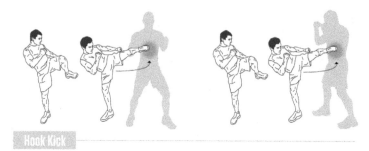

Hook Kick

Lee, Jackie Chan and Jet Li on the other hand use mostly arc kicks. Modern cinema will use arc kicks or jumping push kicks because they are visually more pleasing plus they are a little harder to execute correctly which is why they are more prevalent in popular culture. From a purely practical point of view push kicks tend to be more effective in most unarmed combat situations.

Starting Point

There are two important things to keep in mind when executing kicks. First every kick that requires muscles to coil and spring starts from the same initial position, called "chamber position". Whether the kick starts from the front leg or the back, the chamber position is the same and it brings up the leg in the cocked position, the other leg, acting as the support and balance.

Second, the height of a kick is determined by how high the knee is raised. A lot of arc kicks also require the chamber position to be formed prior to execution as they utilize some of the same muscle groups as a push type kick.

Side Kick

Easily one of the fastest and most powerful push kicks you can perform, a side kick can be thrown from either the back or the front leg, used as a checking kick or an attacking one.

Gets its power from: quads (for a fast checking kick with minimal body movement), quads, glutes and obliques (for a side kick where the supporting leg, spins on the ball of the foot to bring the whole body to bear).

Great for: Checking an opponent's attack. Launching a quick attack. Launching a powerful, deep attack (when launched from the back leg with maximum bodyweight behind it).

Striking area: Usually the edge of the foot (called footsword), or occasionally, the flat of the foot.

Turning Kick

Also known as roundhouse kick. It can be a defensive or attacking technique and can be thrown by the front or back leg. It is an arc kick that performs the leg equivalent of a slap, although a very powerful one.

Gets its power from: Quads (for a front leg kick), quads, glutes and lower back muscles for a kick that utilizes the whole body weight to maximize impact.

Great for: Probing an opponent's guard for weaknesses. It can be used as an attacking kick and it is perfect for setting up an opponent for multiple strikes with the same leg, often at different heights.

Striking area: The instep or top of the foot. The ball of the foot (if you bend your toes back and shape your foot to a 90 degree angle). The shin (a favored Muay Thai kick).

Hook Kick

This is a kick that uses the eccentric motion of the muscles to deliver an unexpected blow that comes in from the blind side (usually). This is usually a kick that's used to attack, rather than defend.

Gets its power from: Quads (for a front leg kick), quads, glutes, lower back muscles and front hip flexors for a kick that utilizes the whole body weight to maximize impact.

Great for: Delivering a kick on an opponent's blind side.

Striking area: The heel or the flat of the foot (for a kick aimed at just delivering sparring points).

Front Kick

The most straightforward of push kicks. It uses the leg's basic mechanical movement to deliver a powerful blow in the shortest line possible, between two targets.

Gets its power from: Quads (primarily), glutes, front hip flexors and lower abs. The hip muscles and glutes if it is executed from a back leg position.

Great for: Delivering a kick in the shortest possible time, when fighting in a forward facing position.

Striking area: The ball of the foot.

Push Kick
Although from a biomechanical action point of view a side kick, front kick and back kick are all push kicks, there is a kick that specifically coils the body's primary muscle groups to utilize the force generated and push through a defense or push an opponent away. The push kick generates the maximum amount of power possible from the coiling of the body's muscles and throwing of a kick in a forward facing position.

Gets its power from: Quads, glutes, abs, hip flexors and lower back muscles.

Great for: Pushing an opponent away, breaking through an opponent's guard, kicking down a door (the action is identical).

Striking area: The flat of the foot.

Axe Kick
An axe kick is an arc king in the sense that the leg undergoes a trajectory in order to generate the power it needs and strike a target. In keeping with the purpose of arc kicks, it can generate a disproportionate amount of power for the muscle groups it uses.

Gets its power from: Front hip flexors, pelvic muscle and lower abs.

Great for: Striking a target with a vertical top-down motion.

Striking area: The heel of the foot.

FIGHTER'S
WARMUP

10 REPS EACH © darebee.com

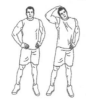

neck rotations

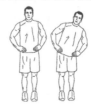

side bends·

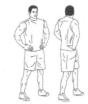

mid back turns

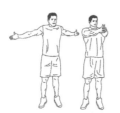

chest expansions

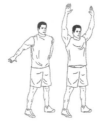

wide arm circles

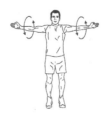

raised arm circles

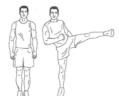

side leg raises

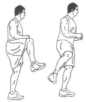

hip rotations

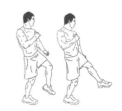

light low front snap kicks

Kick Combinations

Kick combinations are designed to get round the seeming impossibility of delivering successive kicks without compromising one's balance. They are usually delivered in an alternative-legs style so that the body is repositioned after each kick to deliver a new one with the other leg and this minimizes downtime between kicks and does not require extra steps to be taken between kicks.

Different kicks can also be delivered with the same leg, though usually, when that happens mobility and power are sacrificed.

When it comes to fighting kicks are the great equalizer. By using strong muscle groups in the body to attack a target they make up for deficits in strength and reach. A weaker fighter, for example, can overcome a much larger, stronger opponent, by delivering strong kicks at vulnerable areas.

As such kicks are not only the great equalizer allowing, say a woman, to beat a stronger larger man in fighting but also help reduce risk by increasing the safe distance from which you can strike at a target.

How to warm up before doing kicks

Kicks use large muscle groups in fast, explosive movements. Unless you have warmed up beforehand engaging in this kind of activity significantly increases the risks of a sports injury. There are two effective ways of warming up for kicks and both are necessary: First, raising the temperature of the muscle groups by raising the overall temperature of the body. This requires a little light running, jogging on the spot, skipping rope, doing push-ups. Second, raising the temperature of specific muscle groups by increasing the blood flow to them. This requires executing a technique in a powered-down mode, so you are kicking lightly, using the technique to get the muscles you will be using, warmed up and ready.

Getting your kicks right

Power and elegance in execution, in kicks, require good technique. Here are all the elements that make great kicks happen:

- Good balance
- Flexibility
- Tendon strength
- Explosiveness
- Great technique

Good balance requires strong muscles in the supporting muscle groups, not just the ones you use when you perform a kick. A side kick, for instance, puts as much emphasis on the strength and stability of your standing leg as it does on the power of the muscles that execute the kick. Bodyweight exercises, slow kicking techniques, and isometric exercises help develop a lot of the muscle groups you need.

Flexibility is needed to increase speed and free the range of motion of the muscles. There are many different flexibility workouts you can implement here. Flexibility is always a post-workout exercise and some workouts you do should be all flexibility, ones.

Tendon strength exercises are incorporated in many bodyweight workouts. Tendon strength works the front and side hip flexors that are required for the fast execution of kicks. Infinity circles and leg swings help develop the tendons you need and also strengthen the supporting muscle groups.

Explosiveness is developed through anaerobic HIIT training and by pushing the muscles past their limit with exercises to failure.

Powerful Combos

It is always relatively easy to learn to perform a single kick. It takes an understanding of the technique and the power it generates and the development of good balance in order to execute it. Kicks, however really begin to make you feel awesome when you can perform a combination of them in the blink of an eye. That takes a little more practice and it requires an understanding of what goes together and why.

You can't for example, easily use one push-type kick after another. Because push-type kicks coil the muscles and explode in a more or less linear motion, they take some time to get into the starting position so a succession of such type of kicks is hard because it is slow. So one side kick performed after another is self-defeating, just as it is self defeating to perform one front kick after another. The target you're hoping to hit has either moved away in the time between the kicks or, worse, has struck back.

Combinations, therefore, tend to have a very distinctive rhythm of form that looks a little like this: push-type kick + arc-type kick + arc-type or push-type kick or, inverting this: arc-type kick + push-type kick + push-type or arc-type kick. The reason two push-type kicks can be performed together in quick succession at the end of a combination when they shouldn't at its beginning lies in the mechanics of combining kicks. Beyond the fact that a combination of kicks, performed well is great to see, there is a practical reason we do this: it allows us to strike a moving target, using our legs but without taking unnecessary steps which would signal what we do and make it easy to counter or evade and which would also slow us down.

So, an attack combination might look like: side kick + turning kick + turning kick or side kick. After a combination of kicks starts the way it finishes depends on where a target and how fast it is moving to avoid being struck. In the example above, if the target is not moving very fast to get away the combination can finish with a turning kick because the target is within range from the previous strike. If the target is trying to get away however (eg. an opponent back-pedaling) a turning kick is likely to end up short whereas a side kick gives extra reach and can still strike it.

That also suggests how you learn to choose which kick to use in the first instance and when you should sacrifice good balance and mobility and deliver successive kicks from the same leg, without putting your foot down in between. Basically the choice of opening kick is governed by the distance to the target and whether it is moving away as it is struck, or remaining relatively stationary and within steady reach. Facing someone determined to fight with you, for instance, means you don't have to chase them so the kicks will be arc type (unless you want to push them further away from you). If the target is not moving away you can use successive kicks thrown from the same leg (double and triple kicks) and these can even be of the same type and they can be thrown at the same height or varying heights, depending on the situation.

Someone who is moving aggressively towards you, requires a push-type kick to act as a checking kick, quickly followed up by an arc-type kick (as they're not moving away and you do not have to make up for distance).

Putting kick combinations together is a skill and the best way to get better at it is to visualize a sparring scenario and simply drill again and again in a particular combination, until you are proficient. You can then begin on the next one.

Heavy Bag or Empty Air?

The question of whether you should be practicing kicks on a heavy bag or on empty air is the same one that's asked in boxing about bag work and shadow boxing. Both are needed. Each one does something different. Heavy bag work allows you to develop focus and power and also get a feel for the positive feedback which comes from an impact when a strong kick connects. Practicing without a target allows you to develop balance, coordination and speed.

If you're serious about becoming a kicking sensation then you definitely need both. If you're using kicks as part of your fitness training practicing without a bag is good enough. It always comes down to aims and goals which then govern choice. Regardless what you choose you should always aim to enjoy learning to kick well and just have fun.

Whether you learn to kick because you're doing a martial art or are simply using kicks as a way to spice up your fitness training, the results are the same: greater muscle control, enhanced ability and range of movement in your body and a sense that you have shaped yourself to be an instrument of your will. A real living weapon.

Stretching for Strength & Flexibility

Stretching is one of the most misunderstood activities in fitness. Because it is mostly associated with the "bend down and touch your toes" variety of exercise its importance is frequently overlooked and the benefits it can provide are lost.

As muscles grow and as they age, they change. A balanced stretching routine helps provide more even muscle growth along muscle fibers and an increased degree of flexibility, both of which provide a fuller range of motion, greater freedom to move our body as we wish and provide us with more power when we ask it to do something.

In addition to this stretching also helps achieve:

*   Increased flexibility in the joints
*   Better circulation to the muscles and joints being stretched
*   Increased energy levels (as better circulation brings in more oxygen and glycogen)
*   Better coordinated movements
*   Increased speed and power
*   There are seven different types of stretching and although some overlap and some you will probably do a little of as part of your training anyway, it's good to take a closer look at and what they do.

Active Stretching

In active stretching you assume a position and hold it without any assistance other than that of the agonist (primary) muscles involved in that position. In order to hold the body in a particular position the agonist muscle groups need to tense which means that the antagonist ones begin to stretch. Holding a martial arts side kick position, for example, helps stretch the adductors and increases flexibility and kicking height for the martial artist.

Active stretching works because of a physical response called reciprocal inhibition where when one muscle group is tensed and held in position for a prolonged period of time the muscle group opposing it relaxes as there is no need for it to remain tense, and is therefore elongated. You don't need to hold active stretching longer than 30 seconds at the most and in many cases it begins to deliver results in shorter time intervals of 10 – 15 seconds.

Yoga, in particular, uses active stretching quite a lot. Martial artists and ballet dancers also make heavy use of it. Most sports can benefit from active stretching techniques.

Passive Stretching
Passive stretching is an ideal form of stretching to perform with a partner. It requires the body to remain completely passive while an outside force is exerted upon it (by a partner). When used without a partner bodyweight and the force of gravity are allowed to do their thing. Passive stretching is also called relaxed stretching, for that reason.

Doing the splits is one perfect example of passive stretching. By placing your feet as far apart as possible and simply resting your bodyweight on your hips you slowly allow your legs to slide further and further apart naturally. Because passive stretching happens gradually and it requires some time in each position studies show it is ideal for rehabilitating muscles after an injury.

Static Stretching
Static stretching is probably the most common form of stretching and it requires a stretch to be held in a challenging but comfortable position for anywhere between ten and 20 seconds. Because it doesn't push the body to stretch to any extremes it is frequently used as part of the warm-up routine in sports. This has led to the misconception that stretching is required in the warm up in order to prevent sports injuries and that stretching enhances sports performance.

In 2013 three independent studies looked at this from different perspectives. One, published in the Scandinavian Journal of Medicine & Science in Sports found that static stretching carried out as part of the warm up routine contributed to a decrease in muscular performance and introduced instabilities in the muscles which may also contribute to more injuries occurring, instead of less.

The second study published in the Journal of Strength & Conditioning Research found that static stretching carried out as part of the warm-up routine contributed to an immediate decrease in muscular performance. This was further backed up by the third study published in the same journal that found that long-term benefits of pre-workout static stretching were negligible at best.

Isometric Stretching

Isometric stretching is a type of stretching that involves the resistance of muscle groups through isometric contractions (tensing) of the stretched muscles. Pushing against a wall to stretch your calves, putting your leg, straight on a bar and pulling your head down towards your knee and stretching your bicep by putting a straight arm against a wall and exerting force against it are all common examples of isometric stretching.

Because isometric stretching involves a measure of resistance there is some evidence that it helps develop muscle hypertrophy (increased muscle size) when carried out over a prolonged period of time.

Dynamic Stretching

Dynamic stretching uses gentle swings to take the body and its limbs through their range of motion. Because the speed at which dynamic stretches are performed is gradual and the range of movement is within the comfort zone, dynamic stretching is one of the most highly recommended stretching routines that can be carried out as a warm-up.

Golfers, boxers, martial artists and ballerinas routinely use dynamic stretching as part of their preparation routine for high intensity activity. A 2011 study published in the European Journal of Applied Physiology found that dynamic stretching provided increased performance for sprinters and athletes involved in high intensity activity.

A further, independent study, published in 2012 in the Journal of Sports Science and Medicine compared the benefits of dynamic versus static stretching for high intensity athletes and found that those who used only dynamic stretching in their warm up performed better than those who uses static stretching routines. However, those who combined both had a better range of movement (ROM0 overall, suggesting that a mixed routine could deliver superior results.

Ballistic Stretching

Ballistic stretching is a form of stretching that uses bounce and muscle explosion to force a stretch through a range of movement or a fixed position. This is probably the one type of stretching that's got the worst rap from the American Academy of Orthopedic Surgeons who frequently cite it as one of the most common causes of injuries suffered during warm up and stretching routines.

Because ballistic stretching pushes the body beyond its comfort zone it should never be tried without an adequate warm-up. This warning also suggests that to use it as a warm-up is contra-indicatory. Ballistic stretching is routinely used by (properly warmed-up) martial artists, ballet dancers and gymnasts to take the body part its comfortable range of motion and achieve flexibility and range of motion gains.

Studies on ballistic stretching show that when performed post-workout or as standalone workouts it can provide greater benefits in the range of movement and contribute to better performance, something that martial artists, gymnasts and dancers know only too well.

PNF Stretching

PNF stretching which is also known as proprioceptive neuromuscular facilitation stretching, is a set of stretching techniques that can increase both active and passive range of motion and provide real gains in flexibility.

A study published in the Animal Science Journal found that stretching (which includes PNF) can activate the muscle building pathways leading to increased strength and muscle size as long as the stretching is performed after high intensity exercise.

When it comes to stretch routines PNF is probably the king of stretches using resistance against an applied force, followed by relaxation and a repetition of the stretch to achieve rapid gains in flexibility, joint strength by eliciting four separate, sometimes overlapping responses: autogenic inhibition, reciprocal inhibition, stress relaxation, and the gate control theory. All of these are explained in detail in a study on PNF benefits published in the Journal of Human Kinetics.

When Should Stretching Take Place?

If you are using stretching in your pre-workout warm-up routine you should use either Dynamic stretching or PNF, otherwise all stretching should happen post-workout, when the muscles are thoroughly warmed up or it should be a workout all of its own (on a separate day) like the Darebee Stretching Workouts we put together (you can search the site for more).

Studies show that there is no evidence to suggest that pre-workout stretching reduces injuries, on the contrary they show that pre-workout stretching usually affects the ability of the muscles to give 100%. The same studies also show that post-workout stretching and stretching that is part of a separate workout routine deliver greater range of motion benefits and help increase muscle strength, speed and agility.

The bottom line is that stretching is definitely needed and it will always help you achieve more with your body but you should choose carefully when you do it and what type of stretching you do. You can always use a variety of stretching exercises rather than just stick to one particular type of stretching and you should always have some kind of stretching factored in, to maintain the health and elasticity of your muscles.

There are three things that make a perfect fighter and they all work in a complementary manner in the end: Flexibility, tendon strength, neuron density in the muscle. To understand why consider them in reverse order.

Neuron density is achieved through repetition. Repeating moves helps create "form" which is another way of saying muscle memory. This builds up neurons in the muscles being worked that makes them more responsive so they are faster and they are stronger.

Tendon strength is required for execution and muscle stability. When you use a turning kick, for instance, you are partially using the strength of your quads and the speed of your body and your weight but none of that will really help if your side hip flexors are not strong enough to raise the leg without effort. If your tendons are not strong enough the 'heavy lifting' is done by your muscles which means you use up a lot of your strength just to execute each move, dissipating its power.

Flexibility is about degrees of freedom in your body. If we stick with our turning kick example, in order for it to be fast and powerful you also need flexible hamstrings. If your hamstrings are tight you end up using a lot of the power of your kicking leg just to execute the kick so by the time your foot hits its target it hardly has anything left to deliver. Tight hamstrings in your supporting leg mean that your balance is not quite right which will also affect the form of your kick.

Fighters who work on form, flexibility, tendon strength and muscle density end up being in total control of their own body. Ultimately that is what being a fighter is all about. If you do not control your body, there is no hope of controlling anybody else's long enough to beat them.

Fighter's Codex
© darebee.com

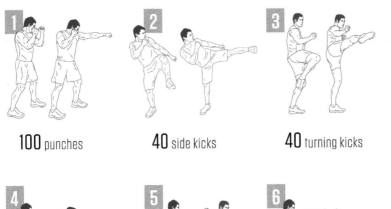

100 punches   **40** side kicks   **40** turning kicks

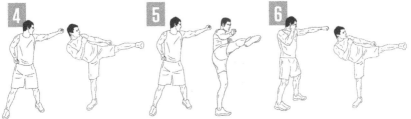

40 backfist + side kick   **40** backfist + turning kick   **40** jab + jab + side kick

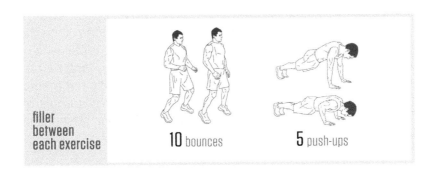

filler
between
each exercise

10 bounces   **5** push-ups

The moment you think of martial arts you think of one thing first: insanely fast punches and kicks. Certainly that is part of it. Repetition of techniques, over time, builds up speed in execution. But that is only part of it. Good fighters are fast not because they can react fast but because they can predict what their opponents are going to do and then move to counter it. Sometimes, the very best fighters, can precipitate an opponent's move by adequately reading them from the start and controlling their movements through an action/reaction plan. But even those who cannot are usually pretty good in seeing what's coming long before it does. It takes a little time and some experience but it's not magic. From any given physical position there are only a limited number of moves that are available and they can be telegraphed in advance by the posture of the fighter. It takes a little practice.

1 minute each | as fast as possible - **1 minute break** between exercises

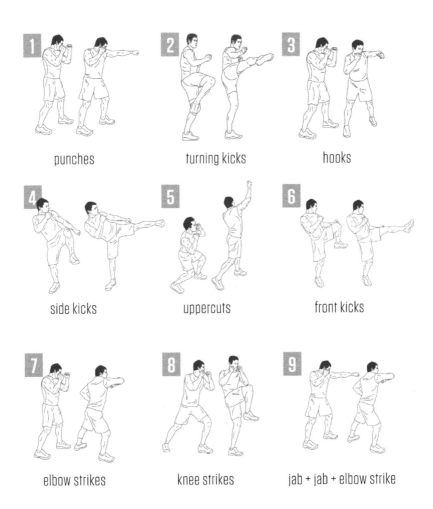

punches	turning kicks	hooks

side kicks	uppercuts	front kicks

elbow strikes	knee strikes	jab + jab + elbow strike

Power has little to do with strength. If that was the case then all martial artists (and boxers and ballerinas for that matter) would have to do is go and lift some weights and be done with it. Power is still a little bit of a mystery, particularly in boxing, where 'heavy hitters' can be surprising. The mechanics that generate it however are fairly well known: you need strong muscles, certainly, but also flexibility, agility, good body positioning, balance and the capability to switch your weight from foot to foot so that your body weight shifts behind your blows. Those who truly think about it, at some depth come to realize that power, real power, comes from the effective use of an attacking limb to deliver the body's weight through an opponent. The limb used is incidental. Once that is understood then each fighter has to work out for himself how to best achieve it within the boundaries of his discipline.

Day 3 | Power

Fighter's Codex
© darebee.com

Level I 5 sets   Level II 7 sets   Level III 10 sets
up to 2 minutes rest between sets

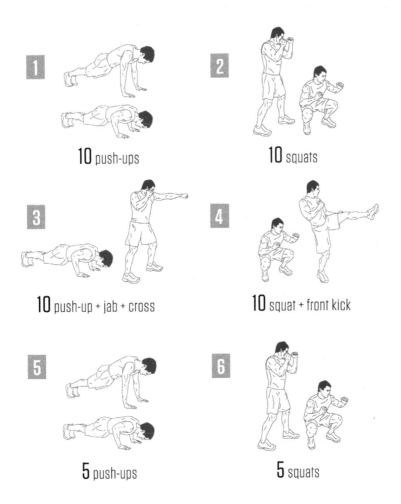

1 10 push-ups

2 10 squats

3 10 push-up + jab + cross

4 10 squat + front kick

5 5 push-ups

6 5 squats

No one really likes stretching. It always hurts. But thinking about stretching as something that needs to be done is the wrong way to go about it. Stretching bestows true freedom of movement to the body. It makes one faster and more powerful just because the muscles can move more freely. So stretching, really, is freedom. And freedom always has a price.

Fighter's Codex
© darebee.com

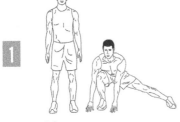

1

40 side lunge stretch

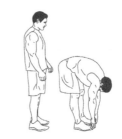

2

20 standing toe

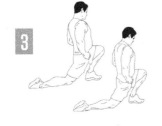

3

40 deep lunge

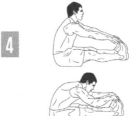

4

60 hamstring stretch

FINISH

2 minute
side split
feet as far apart
as possible

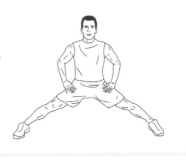

The only way to get good at fighting is to fight. But that is never a realistic proposition. Too much fighting destroys the fighter before he can get good. This is why all martial arts (including boxing) has shadow boxing routines. The fighter there fights against an imaginary opponent. That opponent is perfect, relentless, tireless. The only way for the fighter to beat that opponent is for himself to become perfect, relentless, tireless. Yet fighters are made of flesh and bone. We make mistakes, we hesitate, we get tired. So it's true. The first enemy the fighter has to beat is the only enemy he ever has to beat: himself.

Fighter's Codex
© darebee.com

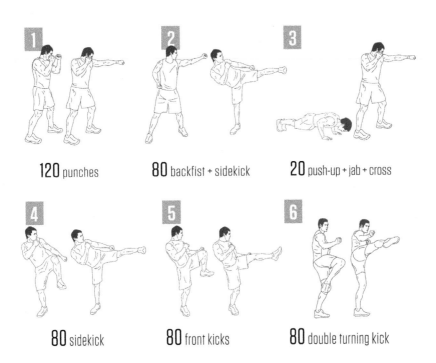

120 punches

80 backfist + sidekick

20 push-up + jab + cross

80 sidekick

80 front kicks

80 double turning kick

filler
between
each exercise

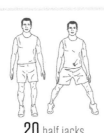

20 half jacks

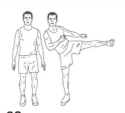

20 side leg raises

The body is just an instrument. When it is trained to perform it can actually do so at will, moving from one motion to another in a seamless ballet of physics and artistry. Martial arts has often been called "ballet with deadly intent". Putting sequences together and practising them again and again allows you to begin to exercise the kind of control your mind needs to have over your body that will transform you into a fighter.

Fighter's Codex
© darebee.com

1 minute each | as fast as possible - **1 minute break** between exercises

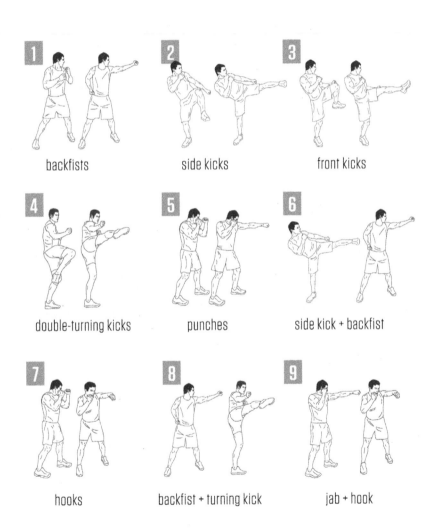

1 backfists

2 side kicks

3 front kicks

4 double-turning kicks

5 punches

6 side kick + backfist

7 hooks

8 backfist + turning kick

9 jab + hook

The body is just an instrument. When it is trained to perform it can actually do so at will, moving from one motion to another in a seamless ballet of physics and artistry. Martial arts has often been called "ballet with deadly intent". Putting sequences together and practising them again and again allows you to begin to exercise the kind of control your mind needs to have over your body that will transform you into a fighter.

Fighter's Codex
© darebee.com

Level I 5 sets   Level II 7 sets   Level III 10 sets
up to 2 minutes rest between sets

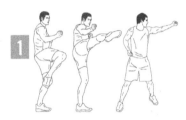

20 turning kick + backfist

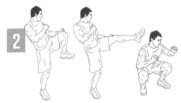

20 front kick + squat

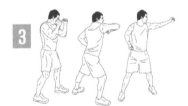

20 elbow strike + backfist

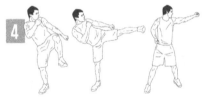

20 side kick + backfist

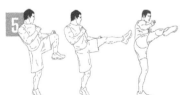

20 front kick + turning kick

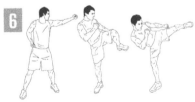

20 double backfist + hook kick

M ost people think that balance begins in the body. You need strong muscles, good flexibility, suppleness and a good sense of physical awareness. Actually balance begins in the mind. To demonstrate the point the moment you shut your eyes your balance is completely destroyed. Balance requires complete awareness of the body and its surroundings. It requires perceptual training which is what really makes a fighter formidable. Balance requires a mind that's truly switched on.

Fighter's Codex
© darebee.com

 1

8 each side + 16 in total
slow side kicks on one leg

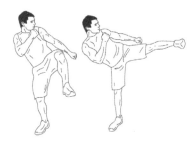

2

8 each side + 16 in total
slow turning kicks on one leg

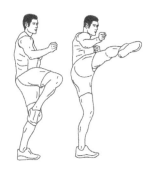

FINISH

blindfold
stand on one leg,
arms out to sides
– then close your eyes
(or use blindfold)

60 seconds

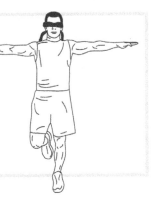

49

M ost people make the mistake of thinking that power comes from hitting hard. It doesn't. A boxer's jab, for instance, is a very hard punch. But it's not a powerful one. Power requires alignment of muscles and a little positioning strategy. Even a light punch thrown against an oncoming opponent can become powerful if he collides with it full force. Power is always the result of a combination of factors that take into account speed, strength, flexibility, balance, position and body weight. Power is what each fighter develops when they begin to acquire their own style.

Fighter's Codex
© darebee.com

Level I 5 sets Level II 7 sets Level III 10 sets
up to 2 minutes rest between sets

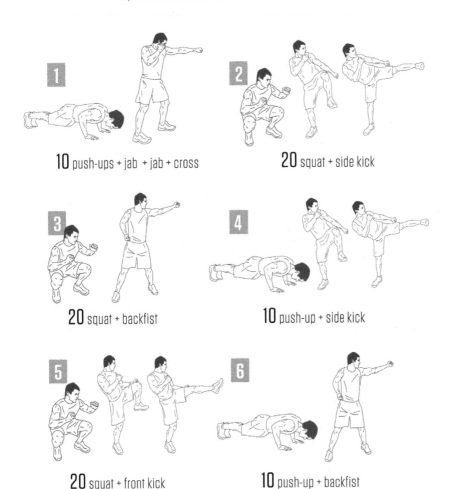

1 10 push-ups + jab + jab + cross

2 20 squat + side kick

3 20 squat + backfist

4 10 push-up + side kick

5 20 squat + front kick

6 10 push-up + backfist

There is something that a fighter always needs to know: where are the limits? What is the absolute maximum of what he can do? Given enough time, patience and discipline there may be no real limits. Maybe the limits of what can be accomplished can only be limited by the limits of what can be imagined. That is a quest that drives every fighter. Always.

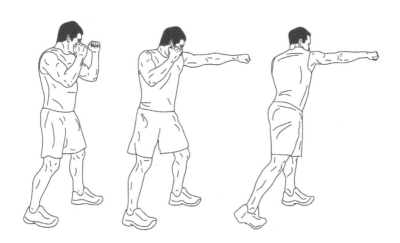

1,000 punches

complete a total of 1,000 punches
by the end of the day

The human body has no claws and no long, sharp teeth. Our upright posture exposes our belly, sternum and throat, points where we are extremely vulnerable. Yet we're not without weapons. The first two knuckles when we make a closed fist. Our elbows, palm heels and knees are areas where our body has a concentrated mass and relatively few nerve endings. This means we can use them to fight back and fight hard. Close quarters combat requires short, sharp moves that are fast and performed in a tight arc with the whole body weight behind them.

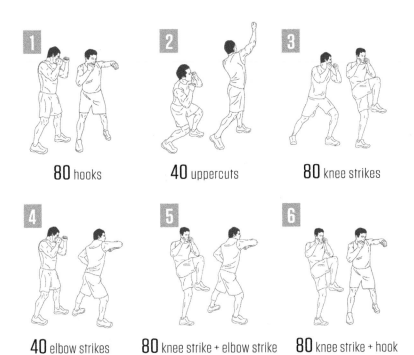

1 80 hooks

2 40 uppercuts

3 80 knee strikes

4 40 elbow strikes

5 80 knee strike + elbow strike

6 80 knee strike + hook

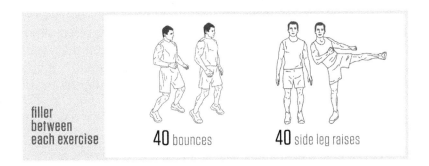

filler
between
each exercise

40 bounces

40 side leg raises

Everyone confuses the idea of a fighter with actual fighting. The body is certainly important. It is an instrument that needs to be fast, strong, agile and durable but the instrument no more makes a fighter than, say, picking up a brush makes a painter. The instrument is just the means through which the real nature of a person is expressed. A fighter is a fighter in their mindset. They learn to ignore setbacks, overcome obstacles, get over difficulties and focus on what needs to be done. A fighter achieves clarity of purpose when almost none is possible. He focuses when focusing is a difficult task. He carries on, when it seems that everyone else is ready to quit. If you're not a fighter in your mind you are unlikely to ever be a fighter in your body no matter how fast, strong or agile you become.

Fighter's Codex
© darebee.com

 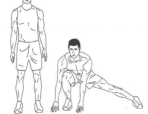 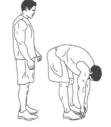

60 side lunge stretch

20 standing toe

 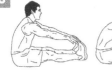 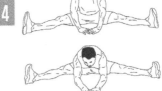

60 hamstring stretch

20 forward bend

FINISH

2 minute
side split
feet as far apart
as possible

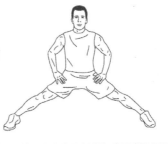

When you punch and kick and shadowbox you have two choices: One, you do everything like you have to but do not feel it. Then every exercise is a chore, every task meaningless, every move without any emotional context. Or two: you can visualize yourself really fighting. You see your opponent, you imagine the moves he makes. In your mind you position yourself to strike and counterstrike. Emotional context makes the moment come alive. It makes your body work in response to a need. It trains your mind to see and adapt. It turns an exercise from a routine to a dress rehearsal. It changes what you do from living to being alive.

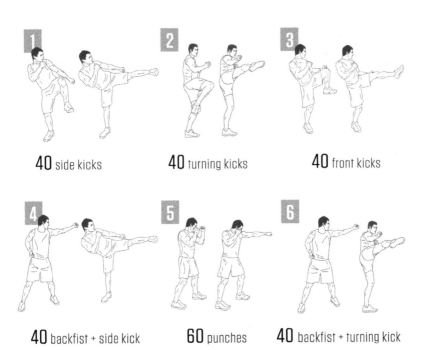

40 side kicks   **40** turning kicks   **40** front kicks

40 backfist + side kick   **60** punches   **40** backfist + turning kick

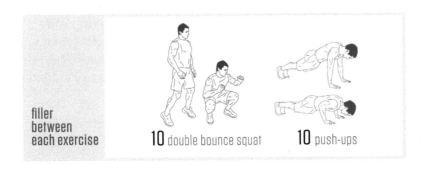

filler
between
each exercise   **10** double bounce squat   **10** push-ups

Although it's not widely known, Chuck Norris took the relatively new art (back in the 70s) of kickboxing to new heights through his synthesis of training techniques more commonly found in sports other than martial arts. He championed bodyweight training, as well as the use of weights for gaining strength and he was a great proponent of long hours of heavy bag work as a means of raising endurance levels. His double-kick combinations in the ring were a new phenomenon at a time when everyone looked for single-kick knock-outs. He paved the way for the open-mindedness that exists in the martial arts world today where training techniques are judged on effectiveness rather than on style.

Fighter's Codex
© darebee.com

Level I 5 sets Level II 7 sets Level III 10 sets
up to 2 minutes rest between sets

1

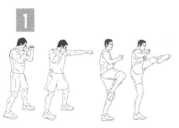

20 jab + jab +cross + double turning kick (mid-high)

2

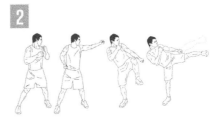

20 backfist + double side kick (mid-high)

3

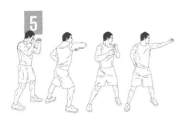

40 double side kick

4

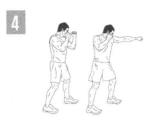

40 jab + cross

5

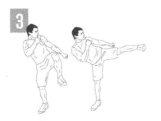

20 elbow strike + backfist

6

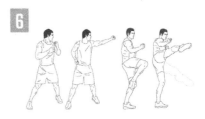

20 backfist + double turning kick (low/mid)

61

Power has a simple enough definition: it is always mass x acceleration. The faster you can hit and the bigger you are the more power you generate. But that's not the whole story. Real power comes from the ability to synchronize your body, using the strength of all the different muscle groups to create harmonious, effortless movements that concentrate speed and strength and amplify mass on small areas. Pushing someone using the entire palm of your hand, for example, is 'softer' than pushing someone using the exact same force but only the front two knuckles of a closed fist. The smaller surface area presented by the latter concentrates the power you can deliver even though the force is exactly the same. Power is all about synchronization of movement, fluidity and focus as well as body positioning and superior adaptive strategy.

Fighter's Codex
© darebee.com

Level I 5 sets Level II 7 sets Level III 10 sets
up to 2 minutes rest between sets

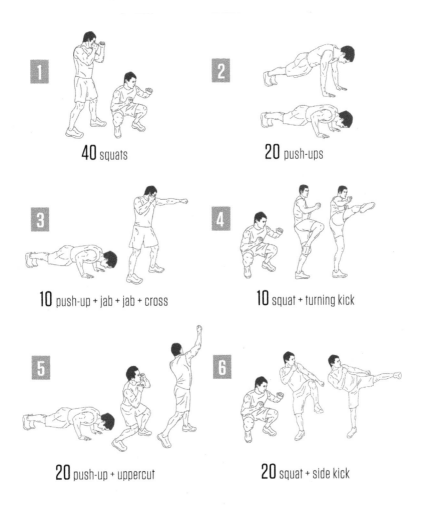

1 **40** squats

2 **20** push-ups

3 **10** push-up + jab + jab + cross

4 **10** squat + turning kick

5 **20** push-up + uppercut

6 **20** squat + side kick

The famous Shaolin Temple monks are probably the best proponents of the importance of balance in martial arts. They spend hours each day practicing balance exercises, forcing their bodies to adapt to positions that challenge them. The reason behind the effectiveness of exercises of balance lies in what they do: they force the mind to find ways to make the body work less though the optimization of stances and positions. This transforms the body into a highly optimized, effective, fighting machine.

Fighter's Codex
© darebee.com

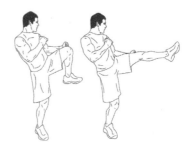

10 each side + 20 in total
slow front kick

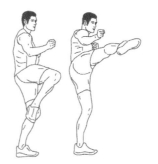

10 each side + 20 in total
slow turning kicks on one leg (high)

FINISH

blindfold
stand on one leg,
arms out to sides
– then close your eyes
(or use blindfold)
60 seconds

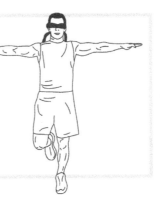

I f you want to become a fighter what's the best way to start? You start
by taking the easiest step. Fighters always play to their strengths. While
you need to work on strength, flexibility, agility, speed and endurance,
positioning and balance your starting steps will be to identify what you're good
at and start using that. If you have reach, for instance, if your arms and legs
are long, it's a good star. If you're strong already you begin to use that. Same
if you're fast. Start with what you're good at and use it as a springboard to get
better.

Fighter's Codex
© darebee.com

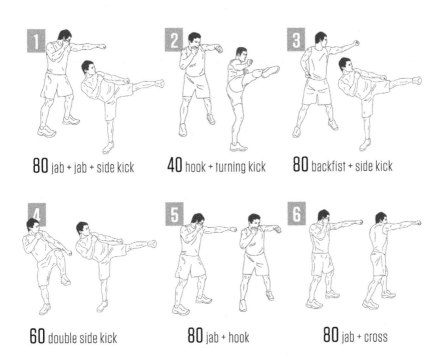

80 jab + jab + side kick

40 hook + turning kick

80 backfist + side kick

60 double side kick

80 jab + hook

80 jab + cross

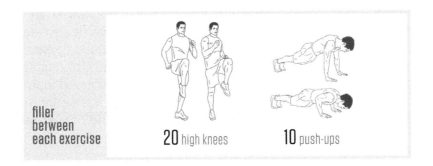

filler
between
each exercise

20 high knees

10 push-ups

Once, a famous fighter in China entered into a fight with an opponent he defeated easily with just three moves. The crowd watching the fight roared their approval and lifted the fighter on their shoulders to parade through the town, marveling at his prowess. Everyone seemed overjoyed at the victory except the fighter. One of his closest friends asked him afterwards what was the matter. He had just won a fight in just three moves, proving how awesome he was. "I lost, today" the fighter replied to his friend. "I learned nothing except how easily the opponent was defeated. I am now lulled into a false sense of security of my own ability that I must break out of. I lost time which I could have put to better use practicing. I have little to be overjoyed about." *Challenge yourself constantly, if you want to get better.*

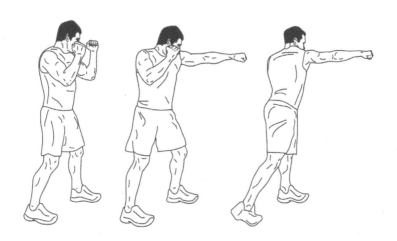

2,000 punches

complete a total of 2,000 punches
by the end of the day

Endurance is the ability of the muscles to work at full power for protracted lengths of time and then recover quickly so they can do it again. Like most aspects of physical fitness endurance is something that can be worked on and improved. Beyond the ability to physically do things endurance plays another role that is just as important. It slows down the onset of fatigue. Fatigue occurs when fuel stores to the muscles have been depleted and insufficient amounts of oxygen are getting through to them. Insufficient oxygen in the bloodstream also affects the brain, slowing down analytical thought. Fighters who have good endurance levels are able to think clearly under pressure. Their brains are unaffected by the demands made of their muscles. They can therefore perform better than untrained fighters.

Fighter's Codex
© darebee.com

Level I 5 sets Level II 7 sets Level III 10 sets
up to 2 minutes rest between sets

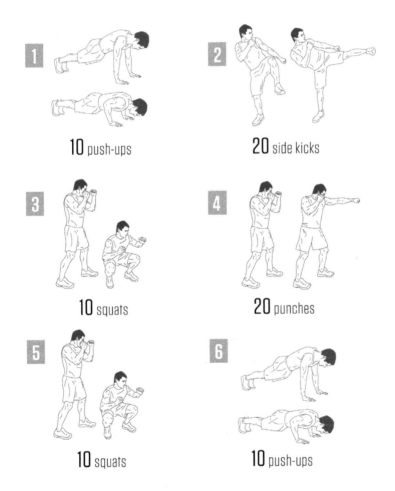

10 push-ups

20 side kicks

10 squats

20 punches

10 squats

10 push-ups

Stretching is a challenge. Every time you are trying to get your muscles and tendons to stretch a little bit more, go a little bit further. This leads to suppleness that helps in the degrees of biomechanical freedom available to you as you ask your body to move. The price you pay, each time is pain. Stretching always hurts, no matter how you do it. There are two ways to get better at this and you will need both. First, the incremental approach. You can get down to doing perfect box splits but it will take time and patience. You simply cannot rush it. So prepare yourself mentally for that and be disciplined enough to actually do it. Second, the habituation approach. In order to get used to the pain of stretching and also see results in the stretching itself you need to get your body accustomed to doing it every day.

If you follow this approach you will find that you do become more flexible, your muscles more supple. Flexibility also helps you become faster as your muscles no longer fight against their own tightness every time you execute a move, which leads to a corresponding increase in power.

Fighter's Codex
© darebee.com

 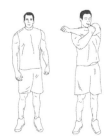

20 calves stretch

 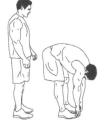

20 standing toe

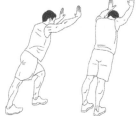

20 shoulder stretch

 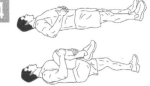

20 knee to chest stretch

FINISH

2 minute
side split
feet as far apart
as possible

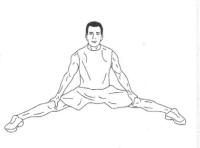

Trained as an artist at the Peking Opera School, a boarding school that taught its pupils operatic traditions of singing, martial arts and acrobatics, alongside their more ordinary studies, Jackie Chan was originally featured in the West as the replacement to Bruce Lee who, at the time of Jackie's first appearance in the West, had only recently passed away. Jackie Chan could have easily taken that path, trying to become a Bruce Lee replacement. Instead he chose to do martial arts films his way, injecting humour and originality in them, making them entertaining as well as thrilling to watch. The point is that who you become has little to do with how you start out. The path you ultimately choose to tread upon is yours, entirely. Find that and you find yourself.

Fighter's Codex
© darebee.com

Level I 5 sets   Level II 7 sets   Level III 10 sets
up to 2 minutes rest between sets

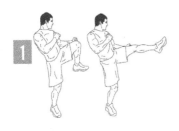

40 front kicks

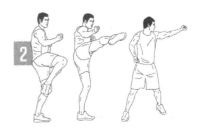

40 low turning kick + backfist

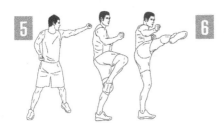

40 double turning kick

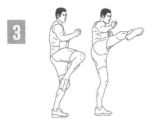

40 double front kick (low/high)

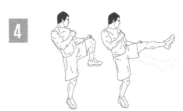

20 backfist + turning kick

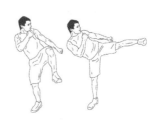

40 side kicks

Training has to be a way of life. The thing to remember is that as you get fitter your body actually wants to do less and less when you really want it to do more and more. This is why it is difficult to maintain the discipline required to stay fit. There is a trick to this every martial artist knows. Before you get into your training for the day start with a routine. It can be anything from basic warm-up exercises to dance moves, jumping on the spot or simply shadow boxing at a very relaxed rate. This is becomes your "key". The moment you start to go through it you take your mind in the headspace required to let your body focus and perform.

Fighter's Codex
© darebee.com

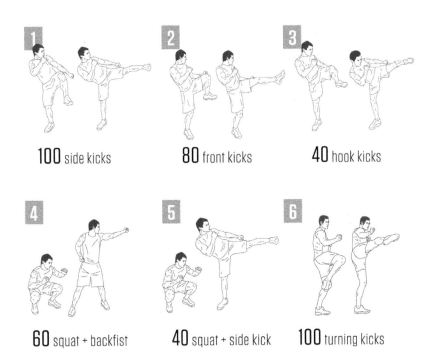

100 side kicks

80 front kicks

40 hook kicks

60 squat + backfist

40 squat + side kick

100 turning kicks

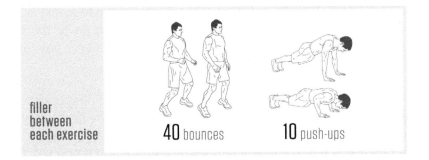

filler
between
each exercise

40 bounces

10 push-ups

We are predators. Our forward facing vision is that of the hunter and we fight our best when we can face our target and use our arms. Despite this the hand is a relatively weak weapon. Boxers and MMA fighters need to tape up their hands to protect them even though they also wear gloves. What saves us, primarily, is that the hand is used to attack relatively soft targets: soft tissue in the body and the chin, temple and nose in the head. Because we have neither naturally hard hands or overly long, really heavy limbs the best way to train is to make sure our arms can move fast, in very precise trajectories.

This is where the Fists of Fury workout helps. By practicing to move your arms fast, even when the muscles are tired you are developing strong muscle memory that leads to fast reflexes and helping to develop the kind of muscle density that leads to punching power.

Fighter's Codex
© darebee.com

Level I 5 sets   Level II 7 sets   Level III 10 sets
up to 2 minutes rest between sets

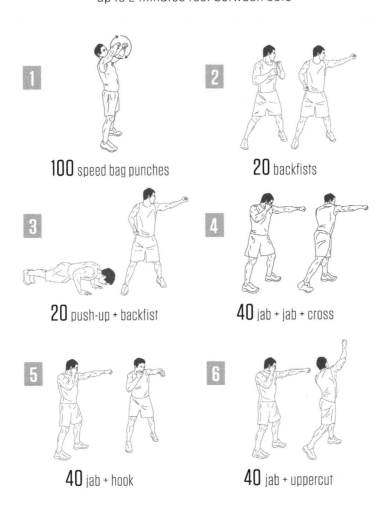

1 100 speed bag punches

2 20 backfists

3 20 push-up + backfist

4 40 jab + jab + cross

5 40 jab + hook

6 40 jab + uppercut

Total muscle control requires superb balance, tendon strength, dense muscles and perceptual awareness of everything that goes into maintaining a fighting stance. Slow execution moves challenge all your muscles and they are a favorite of Shaolin Kung Fu specialists and Tai Chi practitioners alike. The trick here is not to just execute each move but to do so by flexing the muscles involved at the end of each one so that they work, as you hold the move in position, like they would had you executed it fast.

The technique is a favourite one of boxers who execute slow punches this way. It makes them faster and stronger without adding on bulk that requires more energy to carry around during a fight.

Fighter's Codex
© darebee.com

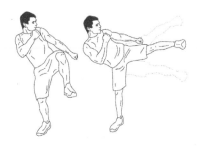

10 each side + 20 in total
slow side kicks on one leg
(low/high/low/high)

2

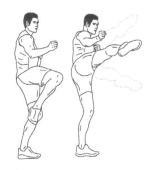

10 each side + 20 in total
slow turning kicks on one leg
(low/high/low)

FINISH **blindfold**
stand on one leg,
arms out to sides
– then close your eyes
(or use blindfold)

60 seconds

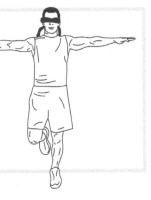

Combinations of kicks and punches are a challenge because they require everything: speed, strength, endurance, balance, flexibility, suppleness, perceptual awareness and good recovery time. The reason they are so good for training however is down to a secret attribute few actually think about: mindfulness.

There is simply no way you can zone out and still perform at this level. When your mind is so actively engaged in monitoring your body and enabling it to move fast and accurately it acts with it as one. It is in the synthesis of mind and body that you get to transform into a real weapon.

Fighter's Codex
© darebee.com

1 backfist +
side kick +
backfist

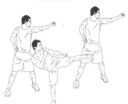

2 side kick +
backfist +
side kick

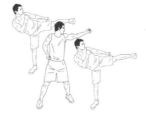

3 turning kick +
jab +
turning kick

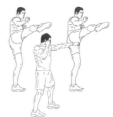

4 front kick +
side kick

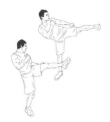

5 jab + jab + cross +
turning kick +
backfist
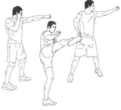

6 jab +
hook +
turning kick
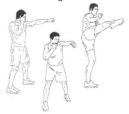

filler
between
each exercise

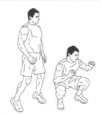
10 double bounce squats

10 push-ups

There is only one sure-fire way of developing speed in martial arts: repetition of précises moves executed at the very limit of one's ability. Speed is acquired by pushing through the limits and the only way to find those limits is to perform as fast as possible to muscle failure, recover and perform again. What happens next is a testament to the body's ability to adapt. As the muscles are asked to perform again and again at top speed for a length of time that challenges them, they change and the limits get pushed further back. If you are serious about becoming the best you can be, seek to find where the limits lie and then strive to get past them.

Fighter's Codex
© darebee.com

1 minute each as fast as possible - **1 minute break** between exercises

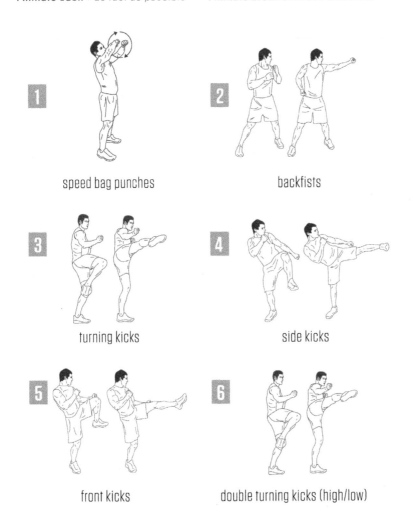

speed bag punches

backfists

turning kicks

side kicks

front kicks

double turning kicks (high/low)

C hallenges require one thing: discipline. Discipline has nothing to do with being regimented or following very specific routines. Discipline is a mind thing. It is the setting of goals and targets and then just getting down and meeting them. The moment something is in our sights discipline is what will help us achieve it. From training to fighting to simply getting through life what makes the difference between having a life and just living is the ability to apply discipline and get things done.

Fighter's Codex
© darebee.com

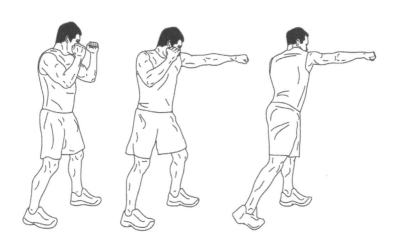

3,000 punches

complete a total of 3,000 punches
by the end of the day

n *The Doctrine of the Mean* Confucius writes: "In all things success depends on previous preparation, and without such previous preparation there is sure to be failure." Today we have popularized this, in the West with "Those who fail to prepare, prepare to fail". This is part of your preparation.

Fighter's Codex
© darebee.com

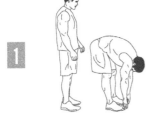

20 standing toes

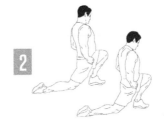

20 deep lunges

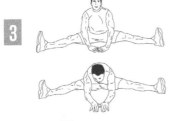

40 forward bend

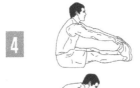

60 hamstring stretch

FINISH

2 minute
side split
feet as far apart
as possible

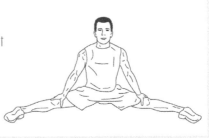

This has been a journey that began with a simple decision: to do the Fighter's Codex, each day, one day at a time. Like most journeys it has been transformative, though to what effect exactly only, the traveller, can say. Some changes happen quickly, they are easy to see. Others are subtle. They happen deeper inside us and are harder to spot. As you are here, on this penultimate day of your thirty-day journey, only you can really tell how much you have changed and how much more you can change.

Fighter's Codex
© darebee.com

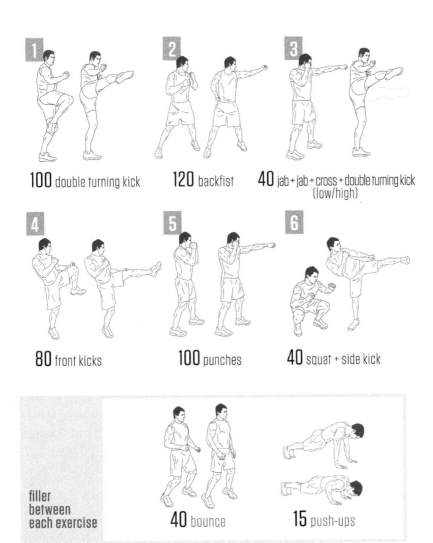

100 double turning kick

120 backfist

40 jab + jab + cross + double turning kick (low/high)

80 front kicks

100 punches

40 squat + side kick

filler between each exercise

40 bounce

15 push-ups

Bruce Lee's tragic, untimely death sealed his stardom in our minds, forever. In his lifetime he succeeded in changing the way martial arts was perceived and in breaking it out of the traditional restrictions that frequently prevented westerners from learning Chinese and other oriental martial arts. In doing so he changed the world, leaving a legacy where the ability to train your body to become fitter was inescapably linked with the need to train your mind to become broader. Throughout this 30-day journey we hope you have felt changes in yourself both inside and out. Maybe, without Bruce Lee, this would not have been possible.

Fighter's Codex
© darebee.com

Level I 5 sets   Level II 7 sets   Level III 10 sets
up to 2 minutes rest between sets

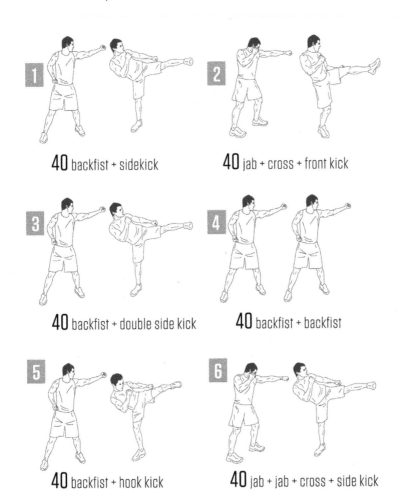

1 — **40** backfist + sidekick

2 — **40** jab + cross + front kick

3 — **40** backfist + double side kick

4 — **40** backfist + backfist

5 — **40** backfist + hook kick

6 — **40** jab + jab + cross + side kick

Fighter's Personal Progress Log

Chart your progress like a professional. Make a note of all the variations you have tried, when you levelled up and what you did differently on particular days where your body performed differently

Name:

Age:

Day Started:

Personal Progress Tracking

Personal Progress Tracking

Personal Progress Tracking

Personal Progress Tracking

Personal Progress Tracking

Personal Progress Tracking

Lightning Source UK Ltd.
Milton Keynes UK
UKHW020707100221
378552UK00012B/1106

Pioneers in Gardening